GAIL FORCE

A MEMOIR OF A
BREAST CANCER SURVIVOR'S JOURNEY

GAIL GANZLIN

GAIL FORCE

Dedicated to all women who have had their breast cancer come back and are now meta-vivors. I pray for your strength and healing.

To my family. Without your loving support,
I would not have made it this far.

To my loving and gracious husband and our two daughters who have
blessed us with five gregarious grandchildren.

To my G-sibs for all your prayers. Even with the geographical distances,
I can always feel your love.

To all my friends who have picked up the pieces of my life. When I needed
you most, you were there for me.

To my oncologist and his team of smart women.
Blessings to all.

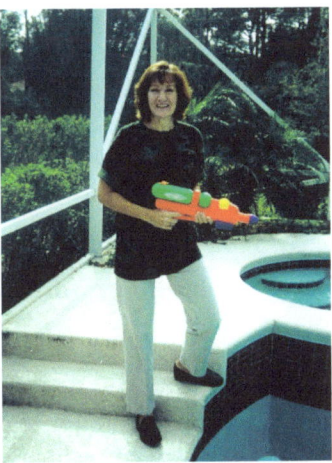

First Day of Chemo in 2000

Bringing Out the Big Guns

I am not a militant by nature; I am from the non-confrontational side of the road. But when slapped in the face at the age of forty-three with a diagnosis of metastatic breast cancer (Stage IV, there is no Stage V), change happens. Suddenly you are fighting for your life.

It all started with a mammogram. I had noticed that my right breast was becoming larger than the left one. My Ob/GYN said to cut out chocolate and coffee, and we scheduled a mammogram for the following month. She had done a physical exam but did not note any lumps in my right breast.

Well besides making me cranky, cutting out chocolate and coffee had done nothing to decrease my right breast. I had the mammogram and it showed I had dense breasts, and they found calcifications. Next was a biopsy, where they cut into my breast and took out tissue to determine if it was cancerous or not. They did not get clean margins, meaning the cancer had spread. After a CT scan of my chest, the cancer was found in my sternum So then they did a needle biopsy of my sternum to determine the type of breast cancer I had. My OB/GYN handed me off to an oncologist. But I was not going to go to just any oncologist; I knew it had to be someone special. I was working my graphic design business and doing a newsletter for a woman and her mother who had beat bone cancer for over 20 years, so I called, told them the story and wanted the name of her oncologist-Dr. H. in West Palm Beach. I would see him.

December 27, 2000. On my first day of chemo I decided I would wear Army camouflage; it was my way of putting my bravest self out there. On the outside I wore a camouflage shirt, and for my head I had gotten a camo cap from my friend whose son was serving in Iraq. Then just some drab khaki pants and some ugly shoes finished my outfit. I cannot remember why I would buy those, much less wear them. Even my granddaughter commented saying, "Why are you wearing Papa's shoes?" This she saw in the photo (page 1) my husband took of me on that day holding a large water gun. On the outside I looked tough (or strange), but inside I was shaking in my ugly shoes.

Getting that first chemotherapy is frightening as you don't know how your body will react. Plus walking into an infusion room is daunting. Where else can you go where people are lined up on recliners, young, old, some with hair, some without? Pink scarfs were everywhere. The feeling of "welcome to your future" surrounded me. I felt nauseous and doomed. I felt my body had betrayed me with this diagnosis. How could it have metasticized to my sternum without my having a clue, other than the slight pain that I attributed to joining a gym the week before? So much for being healthy.

The next five months I was getting Navelbine along with Herceptin and Zometa. Navelbine was the actual chemotherapy drug, Herceptin is an antibody that works on my type of cancer, the Her2nue variety, and the Zometa was to keep it out of my bones. In the beginning I was receiving infusions once a week, but after about a year they changed the protocol to every three weeks. Imagine my relief not to have to put on the happy-I- am- here face every week. I felt gratitude to the drugs for keeping me alive thus far. I received the Herceptin and Zometa combo every three weeks for four years,when after a routine (is there such a thing with cancer?) scan, a spot appeared on my right rib. No biopsy could be taken due to its location. I was back on the chemo Navelbine. As it had worked before, we (I refer to my doctor and me) were hoping it would work again. After eight months of treatment and radiation to the area, the spot was gone, on to living my life.

Before I get too far ahead of myself, let's back up to who I was before I became a metavivor (a combination of words, metastatic and survivor). My husband Michael and I were the parents of two teenage girls, and we had just moved to Florida in 1988 with my husband's job relocation from Wisconsin to Jupiter. We left all our families in Wisconsin where we had grown up in the greater Milwaukee area. How could we pass up getting out of the miserable winters and moving to South Florida? What a gift that move was, and I still love living here today. The nearby ocean is such a peaceful refuge, I try to get there every day.

Once settled, I made the decision to finally finish my BFA degree before I turned 40, and made the drive down to Florida Atlantic University in Davie to take my art classes. In Wisconsin I had worked as a graphic designer at a local newspaper and wanted to continue in that field. I ended up getting a job with a woman that had her own design studio; she was very creative and I learned a lot from her. When she had to move to Atlanta for her husband's job relocation, I decided to begin my own freelance graphic design studio in March of 2000, with the local jobs that did not want to follow her north, but wanted to work with me instead. What a blessing this was for my new business. I had plenty of accounts that kept me busy.

In my personal life, I volunteered at the middle school listening to troubled teens. I was active in the church, I was just a typical suburban mother trying to get the girls through their teen years without my doing them harm. They were pretty tired of my saying "Life's not fair, but God is good." I am not going to get all religious on you, but this mantra, helped with the teenage whining. Things were running smoothly until that day in November, 2000, when after the biopsy the surgeon called to tell me it was cancer.

Whenever a doctor calls you on the weekend, you can bet it is not good news. Being diagnosed with breast cancer is enough to knock you to the ground; having metastatic breast cancer felt like a death sentence. I really did not understand it. So I "googled" it. That was a big mistake. The statistics are daunting and scary as hell. I remember my husband and I were sitting on the bed with tears in our eyes consoling each other and saying "How can this be?" An internal force inside me rose up clearly exclaiming "I will not be a statistic!" I hold on to that truth today, but I have learned "knowledge is power" and to keep on top of the latest drugs for my type of cancer and not to leave it completely in the hands of the doctors. Ask a lot of questions even if some seem stupid. I keep asking till I understand.

I can truly say work was a great distraction. I was working from home and set my own hours. This is also when I became serious about taking care of myself. Our needs come last as most women with a husband and family, and career seem to think, but now that was going to change. The local hospital at the time had a place called the Mind/Body Institute, so I signed up for yoga and tai chi classes. It was the best thing to come out of this bad situation. I continue to practice yoga and tai chi after these fifteen (+) years, even though the Institute closed its doors years ago. I guess they were ahead of their time in thinking Eastern medicine and Western medicine could work in harmony.

Not Your Daughter's Yoga Class

My coping mechanism is yoga. It is what keeps me sane during this madness of cancer. It keeps me aware of how my body feels from day to day. This has helped me stay on top of any changes that may signal a change in my cancer. If you have not tried a yoga class you owe it to yourself to try one, there are lots of classes that do not involve heating a room or turning yourself into a pretzel. There are yoga therapists out there that can teach you poses that work for your particular needs. Yoga teachers are starting to realize that we baby boomers are their future. I have had the good fortune to experience some great yogi's and you always learn something new from each. Coming back to yoga (I had practiced before cancer, but not on a regular schedule) has been an integral part of my recovery. Meditation is also important to calm your "monkey mind"-you know when you cannot stop the thoughts from running wild. One type of meditation concentrates on your breath to calm your mind. I try to do it every day: it is part of my rest. There are lots of good meditation CD's out there, you just have to try some and see what works for you.

Yoga ties into food too, When you are living consciously, you are much more aware about what you are eating - you make better choices. It is a training process not to mindlessly munch. Moderation has been my guide to eating and drinking. Saying no to everything is no way to live, but I do believe that cutting back on diet drinks and extra sugars is important to your overall health, even if you do not have cancer. I personally try and eat all organic vegetables and eat meat sparingly (only hormone and antibiotic free). Thank goodness a Whole Foods opened up nearby and I have a neighborhood organic produce market around the corner. Eating unprocessed fresh foods will make you feel good, and we all strive for that during this difficult time..

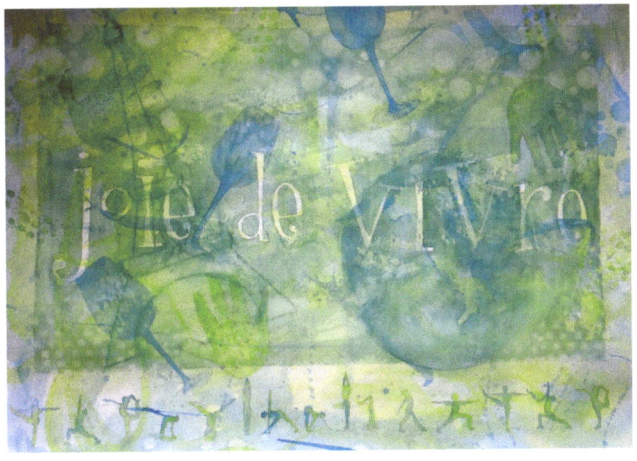

"Joie de Vivre" original watercolor

Cliff Notes

I have not committed all these dates and events to memory. I have kept what I call my "cliff notes" so that I did not have to repeat writing this history every time I saw a new doctor. I would just bring a copy and include it with the clipboard of patient info. I would recommend keeping notes on what procedures and scans you have had. It will make your life easier for appointments with any new doctors. Plus it keeps you on top of vital information that no one else will keep track of for you. I used to write out questions I had for the doctor too, since usually you would forget everything when he finally enters the room. I actually made a little box that I gave to a neurological oncologist I saw up at the Mayo Clinic in Jacksonville. Inside the box I had made little notes that reminded him to "think outside the box" when looking at my case. I tried very hard not just to be a statistic but to make him think of me as a real person with a unique background. Not sure if that made any difference, but it was another way of trying to keep some control in my disease. Everything seems to spin out of control as you try to navigate your uncertain future.

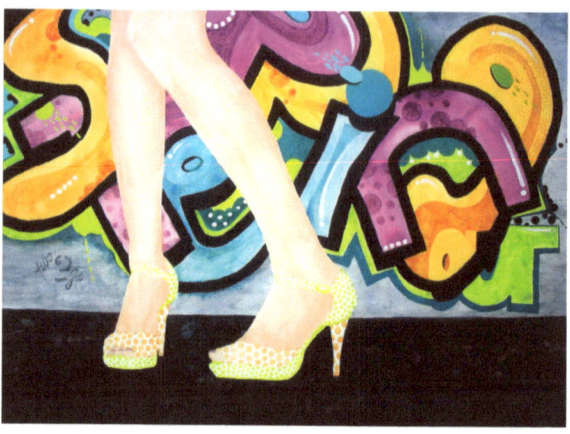

"Stepping out on Wynwood" original watercolor

Music that Moves the Soul

Although I was not blessed with any musical ability other than an appreciation for the music of others, music has always been an important dimension in my life. As a child I had to give up on my organ lessons (yes we had an organ at home) because my ohm-papas would not happen on my left hand while the right hand played the chords. For me music transports my mind to a more peaceful place and moves my soul. Sometimes a good dance when no one is watching is the best medicine. I find I cannot listen to certain songs these days and not tear up. My emotions have been very close to the surface lately. Whatever your style, if it moves you then you need to listen often and dance more.

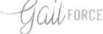

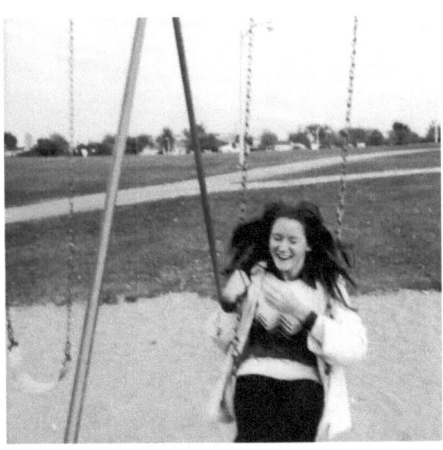

"Swinging Easy" 1975

What Did I Know at 17?

My background growing up, was never dull. I was one of five siblings with names that all start with the letter "G" (I am the oldest girl). Not sure how they decided to name us all with "G's," but I have a feeling it was my father's idea since his name was Gordon and his brother Jerry was naming his whole family with "J"s." I continued the tradition by paying homage to my mother, Mary Lou, and naming my girls with "M's." Melissa and Megan-of course don't forget Michael. My mother was a stay-at-home mom and took care of things on the home front as my father seemed to play the part of Don Draper from 'Mad Men.' We even had a professional hair dryer in our basement. Every morning after he carefully placed a hair net over his coif, he would sit under the dryer till it was well done. He was a successful printing salesman and had the country club membership to show off to clients. I have to say we did not want for anything material. You should have seen the number of presents every year under the Christmas tree. We lived on the northern part of the city of Milwaukee in a one bathroom, three bedroom house for most of my childhood. A second bathroom and additional bedroom were added in the basement, as we grew older and took more time in the bathroom primping. It was the days of staying out till the street lights came on and hanging out with the neighborhood kids. When we were kids, every summer we would all get in the woody station wagon and head east. My mother hailed from a little town in eastern North

Carolina-Swan Quarter. These were memorable trips with my mother in the front seat threatening to hit us with a pink hairbrush if we did not leave each other alone. My father was a driver that wanted you to see what you could out of the window-heaven forbid you should have your nose in a book.

"Look at all you are missing!" Believe me Gary, Indiana is not much to look at. Sure when we got to the mountains, it was a whole lot different. These trips included my younger brother's getting car sick, my baby sister throwing her binky out the window, and my older brother trying to make sure neither I nor my other sister crossed this line he had drawn on the seat. But we would make it to Swan Quarter in one piece, and I have never been as happy as when we crossed over that wooden bridge to my Grannie's house. A group of cousin's would walk to town, which consisted of one gas station, the post office and a general store, to get our Moon Pies and RC colas. Or we'd ride dirt bikes around the big yard, or organize softball games with our cousins. We were carefree, and all the "G's" have fond memories of those long-ago summers.

When we arrived at Grannie's, my father disappeared with my uncle and we would not see him till it was time to go home. We never questioned where they went or what they did. He was not pestering us, and this is when my mother really bloomed. Being "home" with her mom and sisters was when she was happiest. Living in Wisconsin isolated her from her family, and she struggled with depression during the long winters. She had made a choice after meeting this sailor (my Dad) in Portsmouth, VA, where she and her sister were telephone operators. Her other sister married a sailor too, but they settled in Utah near his family.

My mother fought her own battle with cancer as did her mother, my mother had lung cancer that had metastasized, but I was so busy with my small daughters I did not realize it at the time. She had gotten radiation to her brain and now had to wear a wig all the time as her hair refused to come back in one spot. I feel bad that she hid this from us. (Sometimes I think that maybe she didn't hide it, but that I was just unaware.) She survived past five years. Unfortunately, she passed away from a massive heart attack when she was only 57. Her mother had mouth cancer, and the doctors just kept taking more of her gums away, but believe it or not, she still smoked, albeit through a filter device. I remember thinking how this sweet woman was shrinking before our eyes, her mouth held but one tooth and eating was an arduous task for her. We all could not understand how she could still smoke. It is a horrible addiction, and I am glad smoking made me sick when I first tried it in my teens, so I did not succumb to its power. As kids we were exposed to second-hand smoke. But lung cancer can show up even in non-smokers. It is a very hard cancer to beat. I just lost my friend, Carol Ann to it.

The summer I was seventeen, I was working at a place called the "Fruit Ranch"-it was a job my uncle, who was friends with the owners got me and my older brother. I was the candy girl, and $100,000 bars were my favorite, (it was not my job to eat the profits, but to fill the store shelves). My older brother worked in the produce section and worked with a man I thought was at least in his late twenties; he had a full beard, long hair and sometimes had a cigarette or pipe hanging out of his mouth, and his name was Michael. It was customary for the "Ranchers" to get together for a Memorial Day picnic, so I agreed to go with my older brother and his annoying friend. I was in my last week of high school and had plans (mostly made by my father, to go to school in Utah, to study to be an airline stewardess). I was to leave in the early fall. Since it was late spring in Wisconsin, of course it was a nasty day along the shores of Lake Michigan at the park we had decided on for our picnic. There was plenty of beer and fun, and I got to meet the "produce manager" who I had thought was so old. Turns out he was twenty-one and working full time while finishing his degrees in psychology and political science at UW- Milwaukee. We had a good conversation and continued on to a Woody Allen film festival playing at a local theatre. He brought me home and suggested we go to another movie-a real date-sometime next week. I was happy to have this invitation, and got out of the car and headed up to the door of my house. My older brother of course was razzing me about who I came home with. I was so happy to be asked out on a date because I hated high school and all the stupid antics that went on, and I never was part of any crowd, kind of a loner, so had no experience with someone being interested in me.

My self-confidence was below zero (I attribute this to my father who was a very critical man). Michael saw something beyond my low self-esteem; he brought out another side of me I had not realized was there. He listened, I listened to him, we shared some similarities in our upbringing, and we hit it off. Never mind that I was due to leave in a few months to go to Utah to school. He had the saddest look when I told him the plans could not be changed according to my father (remember non-confrontational). My father was anxious to have one child out of the house and on to bigger things. Michael showed up on date night in his silver Chevy Caprice right on time and came to the door, which I promptly answered and headed quickly with him toward the car before any comments could come from the peanut gallery. My mother had a good sense of humor and yelled to me, "Jesus was here" since Michael had long hair and a full beard. She called it right. As it turned out he did save me from the tumultuous relationship I had with my father. Michael's and my relationship became more serious over that summer and we both dreaded when it would be time for me to go to Utah. But I did go, and during that time we spent a lot of time on the phone, writing letters, and sharing musical cassettes. I lasted a long three months before I was headed back to Wisconsin. Michael and I moved in together (it was the mid-70's), and we lived in a dump where we could not even control the thermostat. We had to pound on the wall we shared with our neighbors to get them to turn up the heat. My parents never visited us there which probably was best. We were married in 1977 on Michael's birthday (so he would not forget our anniversary). He has seen me through it all. He is a great father and now a great Papa to our five grandchildren. Making a big decision that early in life, I can only surmise I was lucky-I have been blessed with his love all these years.

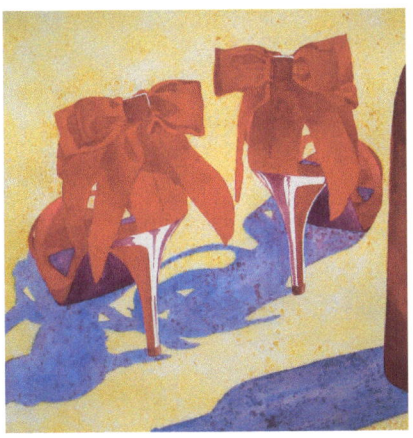

"Reds" original watercolor

The Creative Years

My creativity has been my soul-keeper, my mind-keeper, my sanity solver. I have explored photography, my first college major. Graphic design, my second college major. Then finally I received my Bachelor of Fine Arts degree in 1997. I did not feel my creativity was encouraged by my family. It was more important to study something you could actually make money doing. Art has always been a hard sell, except for graphic design which turned out to be my niche.

Over the years I have pursued other creative endeavors. I created my own line of clothing (named Sugar Magnolia, yes, named after the Grateful Dead song) which I sold to local stores. The sewing of everything myself got to be too consuming with not enough payback. How could I compete with clothing made in India or China at prices where I could see a profit. So I moved on to woodworking and took an evening class at the local high school. I loved the physical aspect and the use of power tools! I started with Adirondack chairs and then designed stools to go with them And a table that could be used between them that I did a mosaic on top. After that I built a tiki bar of my own design that sits on my patio to this day along with my chairs and stools. I also designed and built a floor mirror for my bedroom, which I proudly look upon daily.

My cancer came back, and I could no longer handle the physical attributes of woodworking so I moved on to watercolor painting and joined a group of women that met twice a month for critiques and instruction by Sue Archer, a renowned watercolorist. My artist bio says, "I don't paint still-lifes, but stilettos." I felt a strong attraction to the art of beautiful high heels and painted numerous shoe paintings. Maybe this was my alter-ego coming out. At my age, I could no longer walk in these beauties, but just studying them to paint them was exhilarating. Today I am exploring a new creative side, the art of the memoir. I have never written in my life, so this is daunting territory, but my voice has grown stronger as I progress telling my survivor story. And so it goes...

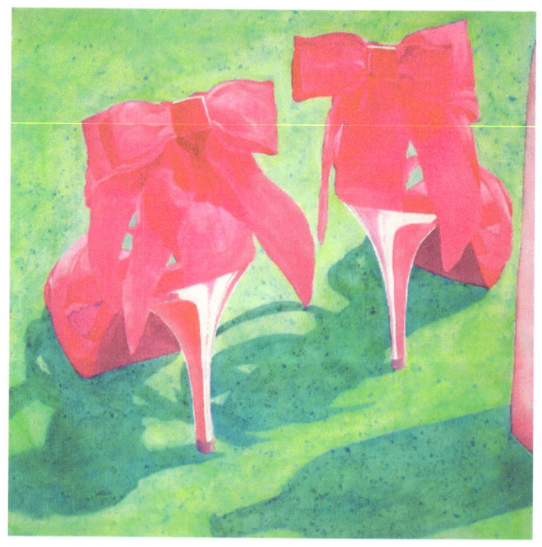

Dedicated to all breast cancer survivors
"Blush" original watercolor

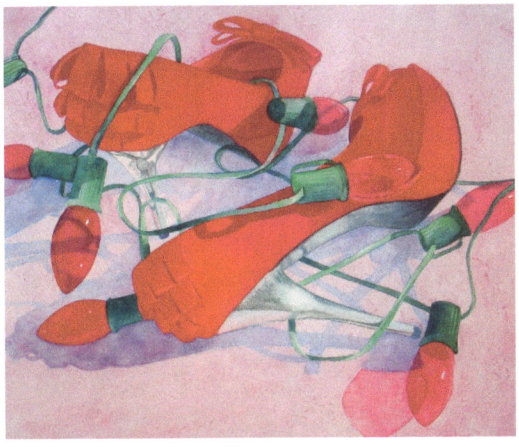

"Is it too late to be good" original watercolor

The Nutcracker

When you get a drug such as Herceptin every three weeks, the doctors suggest you get an IV port inserted in your chest. That way your veins won't give out due to numerous pricks. So remember it was Christmas time when I was to begin my first infusions. I had the port insertion (outpatient surgery), and they had scheduled it for the same day we had tickets to the local production of the Nutcracker Ballet for the evening. I had bought tickets months earlier, as part of a Girl Scout fund-raiser, and I really wanted to go with my daughters to see the ballet before they headed off in their own directions. This surgery was not going to stop me. I had the surgery in the afternoon and was enjoying (despite some discomfort) the ballet that night. I was going to live life like I did not have this awful disease. Denial is a powerful stimulant, and it has carried me through much of what has transpired over the last 15(+) years. It is a survival mechanism that allows the weight of what is possibly my future not to take over. It allows me to stay focused on the here and now. I am mindful every day that it is a blessing to be alive and have the wonderful life I have been given. Now that the port is in place, the next step is surgery.

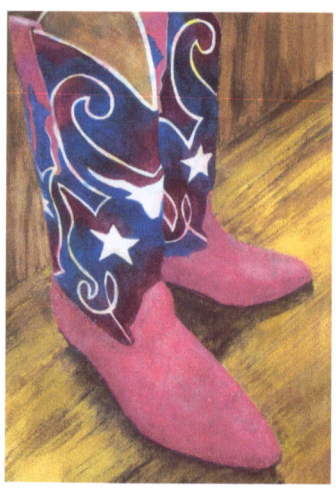

"Texas Two-Step" original watercolor

One or Two Breasts

I was given a choice whether I wanted the one breast with cancer in it removed or both. My first response was, "I don't want this to come back in my other breast. Take both!" Plus I was not too attached to my small breasts-never thought they defined me as a woman. Then I was offered another choice: did I want reconstruction, implants or to go without any breasts, just scars. I chose to have implants. The process, (in the year 2000) the plastic surgeon put in temporaries that would need to be filled every other week with saline to stretch the skin to make room for permanent implants after around three months. This was a painful process, I liken it to when I had braces and they had to tighten the wires. The expansion process was one that I was so happy to have behind me. Now it was time for the perky implants.

Surgery and a Hard Drive Crash

You would think after having this first surgery to remove the breasts and add the temporaries that I had enough on my plate. When I got home from only one night in the hospital, I discovered that my computer hard drive had crashed. I had just started my own business, and I had all my work to date on this computer. My livelihood was held hostage. So I called my computer guy whom I never really had liked and pleaded with him to help. Yes, I did play the cancer card. He likens himself a superhero, so I knew he would come, even though it was Christmas holiday week. He did save the info on my drive, but he was curious to know how this boob surgery went and did I still have nipples. He was not very tactful and I said no, but his question made me realize I was not the woman I had been before. My priorities had shifted: I was more concerned with saving my life, not really with how I looked on the outside.

My femininity was altered. Before surgery I had small breasts with protruding nipples, and I was always trying to cover them up. Now they were gone and there was a sense of loss. Plus it is hard to feel sexy when you have two lumps on your chest that have no feeling. The breast surgeon I had chosen was what I call a "boob man." I had seen his girlfriend and the work he had done on her and felt this is a man who appreciates symmetry. I chose a small set of permanent implants, maybe barely a "B" cup as I did not want to draw attention to my chest. I still have the same implants to this day and am very happy with how they have held up over these fifteen years. Plus, one big bonus is that I didn't have to wear a bra anymore, so I threw all of mine away. But no thanks to Victoria's Secret I missed the sexy bras and mostly how I had felt as a woman with all her body parts. Maintaining my sexual side has been hard on my relationship with my husband. We have tried to maintain our sex life through it all, but it is difficult. I mostly like to snuggle and hold hands and rub my cold feet on his warm legs in bed. Can't you just feel the romance?

Cyber Attack

I remained on the Herceptin and Zometa for four years before cancer came back in 2004. First it was a spot on my right rib that they could not biopsy due to its location, so I went back on the chemo, Navelbine, and continued on the Herceptin and Zometa. They treated this spot with general radiation, a less precise technique that apparently involved radiating my shoulder in the field too.

The next time cancer showed up as a small spot on my right posterior lung in 2007. A new radiation procedure had come out the year before called Cyberknife. They would implant a "seed" into the tumor guided by a CT scan. Once this was in place, high-dose radiation would be administered over three, one and a half hour sessions. As opposed to lung surgery, my oncologist was recommending the Cyberknife treatments Since it was less invasive, with no chance of my lung collapsing, and no post-op. I decided to go with the Cyberknife since it was being touted as the new science of radiation. I had the notion that newer had to be better. It turned out that for me there were side effects from this new treatment that doctors were not completely aware of. I had developed scar tissue, a hard lump where the Cyberknife was targeted, and was told by the radiologist just to have it massaged away which did nothing, Exactly a year after my treatment, I noticed that my right arm would not lift both vertically and laterally. No one ever said it was from radiation, but until I get a better answer I am sticking with my belief that it was.

I saw over fourteen doctors in a year, all trying to figure out why my arm did not work correctly. I had scans and more scans and EMT tests (nerve conduction) and a year of very physical therapy. The best theory they could come up with was that there had been an injury to my brachial plexus: the nerves in the shoulder of the arm must have been damaged by an earlier radiation that I had had for the rib metastacist in 2004. Who do you hold accountable for a procedure that has saved your life but left you with a disabling side effect? I have had to adjust to being mostly left handed-where there's a will there's a way. It did not keep me from holding my grandchildren, and for that I can't complain, I have to remain grateful for my longevity.

Freakin' February in Minnesota

In this chronology, after seeing so many doctors, my husband and I spent a good deal of time online to find a doctor who knew what he was talking about. In February of 2008 we came upon a link for a brachial plexus clinic at the Mayo Clinic in Rochester, Minnesota,. There was a neuro-surgeon on staff that looked promising. Maybe he would have some insight as to why my arm was not working. You probably think me insane by now, but going to Minnesota in February was really nuts. The temperature was reading -18° on the bank sign in downtown Rochester, but the good thing about the Mayo Clinic up there is that everything is accessible underground. It is a beautiful facility with artwork on the walls, a grand piano playing, a great cafeteria, but it still felt institutional and huge, and I got the feeling I was just a number. We saw the doctor after another round of MRIs. They were looking at a lesion (they thought was cancer in between my cervical spine C4-5). My first impression of this surgeon, was apprehension (my gut talking to me again). He sashayed into the room with an intern taggin' behind him. He suggested we do exploratory surgery on the nerves between my shoulder and neck. A red flag went up for me, and we asked what was the risk? Casually, he said, "Maybe loss of any movement in the arm." But he was sure it would not come to that, and he was sure there was cancer hiding in them there nerves. As we finished our consult and he was leaving the room, he karate-chopped me on that side of my neck. No explanation. He was out the door. I was stunned as was my husband, and we walked out of there even more confused. Over dinner that night, (underground Italian), we discussed what had transpired. When we got back to the hotel room, we canceled the 6 am surgery. Got on a flight the next day back to warm Florida.

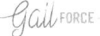

Practicing Medicine

For eight and a half years I took a bone strengthener called Zometa. I got this drug along with the Herceptin every three weeks. I had been reading the Team Inspire website, a great resource for women going through metastatic disease. I started doing research on this drug. The protocol was for it to be given every three weeks, but I could find no reference on the manufacturer's site as to how long it should be given. This was new territory even having survived this long. I had seen a bone specialist and got no answer from him to explain the spots on my bones that were showing up on scans. My regular oncologist did a couple of needle biopsies, one on my hip and one I particularly remember on my sternum. My onocologist had to practically sit on my chest while he stabbed me with a needle. I remember looking at his nurse and she had this look on her face revealing how bad she felt for me. I had to call my sister after that and have her meet me for a beer. But these needle biopsies never showed a trace of cancer.

This time I went to the Mayo Clinic in Jacksonville, Florida. No more Minnesota. After many tests and a spinal tap, they determined I had a lesion in my cervical spine between C4 and 5. They scheduled radiation to be done at my local hospital. I had been having neck pain but thought it all had to do with the bone strengthener. Apparently it was unrelated, the local radiologist had his reservations about doing radiation to my neck without having a biopsy, but it was determined up at the Mayo by their doctors that it was too dangerous an area to biopsy. Having radiation anywhere on your head or neck necessitates having a mask made of plastic mesh that they clamp to the radiation table so you cannot move. Luckily these treatments were very short, and I usually only made it through a couple of my Dr. Seuss mantras. One cell, two cell, three cell - four, five cell, six cell, seven cell more, eight cell, nine cell, ten cell: DEAD!

I had six weeks of daily (M-F) radiation to my neck. At the end my neck pain was gone but I still had to take chemotherapy for six months. I was still experiencing pain in my right hip and leg and saw an orthopeodic specialist up at the Mayo in Jacksonville who referred me to a phsyiatrist, which is a rehabilitative doctor. He came in the door in a wheelchair, and we discussed my issues with my hip pain. He went over to a corner of the room and handed me a cane! Here is the answer to your problems, I almost took that cane and hit him over the head with it, but since he was already in a wheelchair, I just could not do it. I walked or hobbled out of there disappointed again. Why was no one mentioning the bone strengthener and the research I had discovered on-line about how this drug not only causes necrosis of the jaw but was showing up in fractures in femurs. The stories I had read on the Team Inspire site told of ladies who had been on Zometa a long time too and were breaking their femurs, not from skiing downhill, but just by doing everyday stuff. I soldiered on and kept up my walking routine, a couple miles on the beautiful beach here in Jupiter.

The particular area I walked was usually isolated, but it was a designated dog beach, so when you did see someone they usually had a dog along and not on leashes. One day I had my headphones on, enjoying the day, when all of a sudden two yippy little dogs come barreling down the beach and knocked my feet out from under me. Splash! I landed in the water. The owners quickly came to help me up and apologized profusely. I stood up but my right leg burned with pain, "I'm fine," I insisted (so typical of me). They continued on down the beach. I realized I was about a mile down the beach from my car, and I started heading back that way while crying and limping. Sure enough, an x-ray later that day showed a hairline fracture in my right femur. Now whether this happened that day or had been there before, discovering it had me more miffed because I had received many MRIs of my leg and hip in the recent past. But all it took was a simple x-ray to show a fracture.

Now you cannot tell me that cancer is not big business. They can charge a whole lot more to my insurance company for an MRI. This confirmed my suspicions about the bone strengthener: it was the culprit in my bone pain, not cancer. But at this point since they could not determine what the spot on my femur was, they were going to radiate my leg. As I write this, I realize how crazy this sounds, but I was scheduled for radiation at my local hospital: they had already put the tattoos on my leg (these are just little dots they use as markers). I was scheduled for the next day, but to my surprise I received a call from the doctor who runs the place where I get my MRIs done and he said, "Do not do the radiation. It is not cancer in your leg." "Finally someone gets it!" I thought. He informed my radiologist and oncologist. Saved by a day from being radiated again, I was thrilled. For the fracture, I just had to take it easy and do some rehabilitation while it healed. When people say doctors are "practicing" medicine, I know exactly what they mean. I don't have an M.D. after my name, but I have earned a H.K. It stands for Hard Knocks.

I was about at my wit's end. When I was seeing another doctor in Miami, he said, "Has anyone told you have Horner's Syndrome in your right eye?" I had never heard this from my oncologist. What was it? I have to say it was at this point that I gave up on my then oncologist. She was missing too much information. (I still feel bad when I see her around the treatment center for not giving her a reason for my switch-hey remember non-confrontational?) I went back to my original oncologist whom I had given up on in 2005 when I could not get an appointment with him because he was taking care of his son who had cancer. (I cannot blame him for that.) Now I have been with him for the past ten years. Horner's syndrome, it turns out, is having a drooping eyelid due to sympathetic nerve damage. It was another thing to add to the damage I suspected the Cyberknife had done. Of course no one points any fingers or gives you direct cause and effect, but my drooping eyelid symptom did not appear out of nowhere.

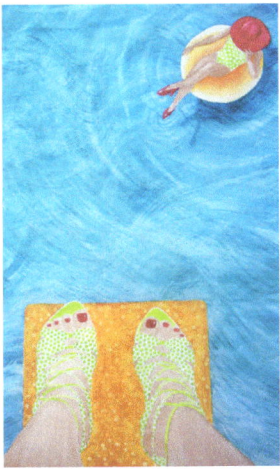

"Swan Dive" original watercolor

Leap of Faith

June 11, 2009, was my day of clarity, I don't know why it happened then, but I knew what I had to do to save my sanity in this cancer mess. I declared to my doctor that I wanted off all medicines to give my body a break. Eight and a half years of toxic assault on my body had my mind fighting back. I did convince my doctor that this was my wish, and he understood, since he could not give me any evidence that being on these drugs for so long had been in my best interest. I thrived for four years, not worrying about going in for infusion. It was during this time that I learned my oldest daughter was due to have twins in the fall. It was also when I could help my step-mother take care of my father. As his health was failing and she wanted to attend a family reunion, I was able to spend time with him before he passed away. Having the time to help my daughter and then son-in-law was such a blessing for all of us. Raising twins is hard, and they had tummy problems that kept us up during the night so we took it in shifts, and I was feeling great during that fall. My husband and I were able to plan that trip to Ireland we had talked about, but we should not have gone in May when the rain came down horizontally and it was cold. We enjoyed the tours and the Irish pubs. I was actually putting cancer behind me, and it was so freeing.

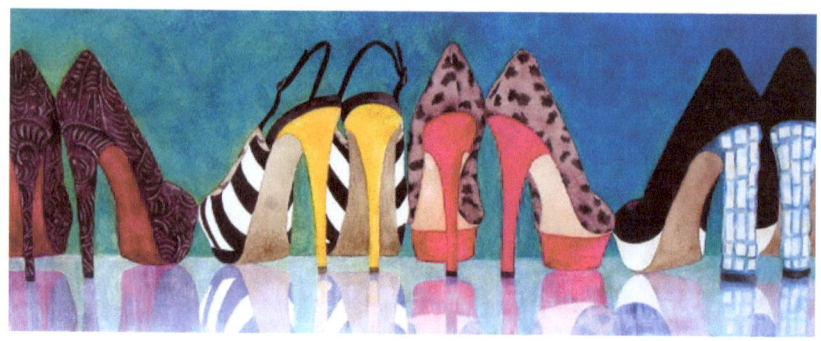

"A Shoe for all Reasons" original watercolor

Terrorism

It was a great four years and I do not regret my decision. Hey, this cancer is sneaky and it will come back whenever. So why not live your dreams? Sneak attacks reminded of that horrific day, eight years earlier, in September. I would not have known what was going on had I not been in my yoga class and the World Trade Center was on the TV at the gym. Everyone was watching. I stood in disbelief at what I was seeing. We continued yoga class and practiced our mindfulness while we prayed for the victims of 9/11. I realized that I had been living with a terrorism threat named cancer. It compared nothing to the destruction that appeared on the TV screen, and even though I did not know anyone personally that perished that day, this event scarred our country and still does today. I curse the terrorists every time I have to take my shoes off and go through the TSA line at the airport.

Breath of Life

In 2013, another personal terrorist attack came after I noticed a shortness of breath in my yoga class while doing a pose called downward dog. I called my oncologist who had me seeing a thoracic specialist by the end of the day. He proceeded to drain 1.5 liters of fluid from around my right lung. I joked with him, 'Do you have a keg back there?" Since the fluid looked like beer.

Again my body had betrayed me, I had no idea about this invasion as I had just walked three miles with my girlfriend that morning and had been able to hold a conversation. The terrorist had moved into lymph nodes above my right lung, and the fluid was filling the sac that envelopes the lungs so they can move when we breath. It is called pleural effusion. I had a catheter which I had to drain twice a day placed in my right side for three months., The fluid was supposed to dry up from the chemo I was on. Every time I drained the tube, I prayed the number would get to a level that nothing further would need to be done. But no, it decided to be stubborn and hang on, and now I was headed for a procedure called a pleurodesis. This was during the summer, and I had planned my mother's side of the family's reunion to be held in July in eastern North Carolina. There was no way I was missing that, so I went and kept what I was going through to myself. Sometimes it is easier to bear than trying to explain the details most people would not understand. Sheer determination got me through that tough time.

When I got back from my reunion in N.C. and the amount of fluid was still too high, I was scheduled for the pleurodesis. They neglected to tell me that I would have a chest tube and would have to stay in the hospital until it drained almost completely. That turned out to be six days. The worst of it was that they had put me in a room across from the emergency entrance. I had trouble sleeping through the sirens. Finally on one busy Saturday night, I pleaded with the nurse to give me something to help me sleep but she only had orders for Benedryl. It helped, but I think I have post traumatic stress syndrome because I cannot go by that part of the hospital without feeling sick and remembering that horrible stay. I made sure to tell my oncologist that if I ever ended up in the hospital again, he'd better put me in a room that overlooks the intracoastal waterway and the island of Palm Beach. Such is the life here in Palm Beach County.

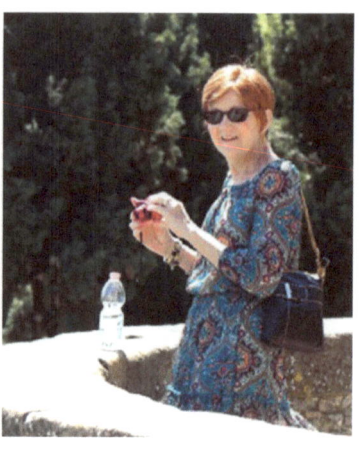

"Buongiorno" 2016

Lucky Me - Italy!

I love to travel. When I was dancing with N.E.D. (No Evidence of Disease) again after my lung recurrence, my best friend Deb and I decided we were going to travel somewhere. Not sure where initially, we were both keeping our eyes out for something interesting, and we both found it about the same time. An ad on Facebook read, "Ignite Your Bliss" a yoga/photography retreat in Tuscany, Italy in May of 2014. We would do this!

We had to book a flight to Florence. I was coming from West Palm Beach and Deb from Santa Fe, so we would try to book a flight from NYC to Florence so we could fly together. Unfortunately our schedules did not sync up, and we ended up flying on different flights from NYC. My layovers would be Atlanta to NYC then NYC to Paris then on to Florence. She was going to do a red eye out of Albuquerque to NYC then a layover in Zurich then on to Florence. Her flight was uneventful, but mine took a turn in Atlanta. The plane was in a long queue to depart, but I could see dark clouds on the horizon. Praying we would beat the storm and get this long flight on its way, we had sat on the tarmac for over an hour when I noticed the plane was moving back toward the terminal. It had not starting raining yet, and I was wondering what was going on. The pilot came on the PA and said we needed to refuel because of having waited so long, and we would now wait for the weather to pass before we got underway. When faced with an eight-hour flight, this is not what you want to hear. Now my chances of making my connection in Paris were bleak, and sure enough, when I finally got to the gate in Paris after running what seemed a couple of miles in the terminal, my plane had left. Another plane was to leave in about an hour, so that was not too bad, but I had to text Deb as the retreat coordinators had scheduled a driver to take us to the villa from the Florence airport along with two other ladies. I was exhausted by the time my flight landed- had not slept much. Deb was there waiting along with the other two ladies and the driver of the van. Then, of course, my bag did not make the flight out of Paris, so I had to fill out the forms to have the bag delivered to the villa; it was a weekend and it would take three days to finally get it. Luckily I had packed one pair of underwear and a travel toothbrush. There are a lot of pictures of me wearing the same clothes and, more importantly to me, no make-up. Ugh! It was a long day; a glass of wine and I was ready for bed. Sometimes the odds are stacked against you, then you have to pull strength from within and conquer the problem. No make-up- ha!

The next day we enjoyed a day of yoga and relaxation and started our photography workshop. The photography instructors were a married couple, Gary and Julie, who run a photo studio in Orlando, Florida. They were very good at showing us how to get the most out of our cameras with individual attention. We practiced by photographing the beautiful surroundings. The villa sat on a small hill that overlooked rolling hills in the distance. There are two buildings made of rustic stones: one was our rooms, the other was the kitchen and covered patio dining area with an upstairs that we would do yoga in if the weather was too cool to do it outside. There were beautiful roses growing on the stone walls, and trellises with flowing vines-lots of material for our photographic endeavors. Deb and I shared a nice room with lovely views and a bathroom with a bidet and European shower stall, meaning there was just enough room to pick up soap if you dropped it, but not much more space. Everything was clean, and we were comfy in our twin beds. They had planned excursions out to wineries and sightseeing, that kept our days full. The food at the villa was cooked by a lovely Italian lady, Allesia, who spoke no English but cooked exquisite meals - from homemade cakes for breakfast to wonderful and fresh meals for dinner. Lots of locally grown vegetables somehow tasted better in Italy than anywhere at home. Maybe it was the wine. Of course we used the wine as an excuse to not do yoga in the evenings too. In Italy dinner was usually at 8pm and by the time we were done, we could not get ourselves on our mats, we were ready for bed. We did do yoga every morning, either inside or out. The teacher was also the coordinator of these retreats, and her style was relaxing and rejuvenating. The days flew by all too quickly and before we knew, it we were saying ciao and headed back to the Florence airport.

Since I had such a good time in Italy this first time, I decided to do two more weeks in 2015. I had to book this trip scheduled for May early and had no idea I would be recovering from whole brain radiation (more on that later) again in February. But as the saying goes, "When there is a will, there is a way."

It got complicated as it got closer because my husband did not want me traveling that far by myself. Luckily I have my friend Kitty who at the time was going through a bad divorce and wanted a get-a-way. She no longer had work obligations and was ready to go in a heartbeat. The complicated part was that when I was arranging the flights, I screwed up because of the overnight flight: we ended up spending two extra nights, one in Milan and one in NYC. I had it in my mind that traveling by train from Milan to Florence sounded like a good idea. But with my mind still in flux from the radiation and the steroids, all the pieces did not fall into place. I was trying to arrange for us to fly together and sit together, Arranging the seating was a nightmare with Swiss Air; we ended up paying for seats together, but when we got our boarding passes, we were apart. Same thing on the way back, but we had a kind person who exchanged seats with me so we could sit together.

Taking a train from Milan to Florence was not an easy task for us. It was hard to figure out the train platform system and how they changed numbers on the arriving and departing trains. We did manage to find our way to Florence in our pre-registered seats and were proud of ourselves. The driver of the van was waiting along with the other attendees of the retreat. One was standing in "tree" pose with the group so we could identify them. We all filed into the van for the long ride to the villa. We introduced ourselves to the other ladies and one lone man who had come with his girlfriend who was teaching the writing workshop. He also taught yoga. Once at the villa the coordinators unloaded our bags and took them to our rooms; Kitty and I would share the same room that Deb had the previous year. They had also set out food: olives, bread, cheese and of course, wine to tide us over to our special dinner. The ladies were a boisterous group who knew each other from the Tampa area, and dinner turned into hours laughing. Jet lag can really mess you up, not to mention my low energy level, so it was hard to keep up and stay up late. Kitty was wonderful about helping me, carrying things for me, sharing her hot water bottle (I was always cold there). She even shared her cashmere sweater too. The temperatures were definitely cooler this year than the previous year, we were lucky there was rain on only one day. The first week we enjoyed yoga, excursions to nearby wineries, such as Pienza & Poggio, fabulous meals, and I was learning how to write. We also visited San Gimignano along with a fabulous trip to San Galgano (a monastery that dated back to the 1400ís). It was a glorious week, so relaxing. Before we knew it, it was over and we were saying ciao to our new friends. One big surprise was that Melissa, our writing instructor, who had brought her boyfriend who was also a yoga instructor, got engaged! They had their engagement photos done right there by the photography instructors. We all could see this had been well thought out due to the clothes they wore for the photo shoot. Only a surprise to us!

Week two was the photography workshop, and it was great seeing Gary and Julie again. This time they brought their 3 month old daughter with them. She was adorable, and so sweet tempered you did not know she was there. She also joined her mom on the yoga mat. She just put a smile on everyone's faces. The week was filled with photo shoots, visits to a couple, different than the week before wineries, and back to San Galgano. We were instructed how to handle the partly sunny light with our cameras to make the most of our photography. This place was amazing: the walls were still in place, but the ceilings were all gone so the light played against the stony walls. I have two photos of this beautiful place that I blew up and had printed on canvas and that now hang in my dining room. They always make me think of the song "Happy" ("a room without a roof," is a line from the song). Being immersed in Tuscany was one of the best travel decisions I have ever made and the best healing retreats for my slowly increasing platelets.

Hard to believe our two weeks were done, and we were packing to leave on the van back to the train station in Florence. Unfortunately our van driver did not know where the new train station was located, and traffic was horrendous, so every time we turned a corner thinking we would see it, we just turned into more traffic. When we had left the villa, we had plenty of time to make our train, but as the minutes passed in traffic, we were running out of the luxury of time. Bam, back to reality! Kitty finally found the station on her phone's GPS, and finally we were pulling up to it. We hurried to the platform only to be confused again by the numbering system: the number posted was different from the one on our tickets, although the destination was correct. Kitty was hungry so we ran into a little shop that made sandwiches, but you had to buy a ticket first, then stand in line to get a sandwich. Time was ticking in my ears, and the hustle and bustle was wearing my nerves thin. We ran back to the platform just in time for the train to arrive, and we searched for the coach number our tickets said we were on.

We knew our time was limited, so we just decided to go for any coach and then we would walk from car to car, rather than miss our train. Well, that was our plan, so Kitty threw my purple bag in a car and was about to throw hers on when the doors closed on the train. We frantically pounded on the door, to no avail. They do not have any assistants that are on the platform to help. We were screwed. A nice gentleman from behind us saw our predicament, pulled us back from the departing train, and suggested we go to the Italia office in the train station. We did exactly that and told the woman behind the counter our story. We both noticed the smirk on her face, and we both started laughing. She radioed to someone on the train to let them know of the purple bag. In a few minutes she answered the radio that they had found it and it would be waiting for us at the Florence train station. Whew, but now we had to book another train, and of course we had to upgrade to first class coach, as that was all that was left available. Luckily it would leave in an hour. All the money I thought we had saved on the less expensive flight from NYC to Milan, was now adding up to be more than just going directly to Florence would have been, plus with the two additional nights of lodging, I had totally messed up our savings. Oh but what an adventure! Kitty was very understanding and she held herself partially responsible for not really keeping on top of the details of this trip.

The story does not end there.

We had a nice relaxing ride in our first class seats on the train, shared our sandwich and were feeling grateful for the fact that my bag was safe. We must have been distracted when the train stopped, but we thought we were at the Florence station as so many people were getting off. Turns out once we got in the station, we realized it looked nothing like we remembered the Florence station looking like. We had gotten off too soon. We saw the Metro station and decided to ride the rest of the way by metro. This was Kitty's idea, I am so directionally challenged that if left to me we would end up in France. Kitty used to ride the metro in NYC, so I followed her lead. We bought tickets, and hers worked at the turnstile-mine did not, so I slipped through. We sat on that metro for almost 10 stops before we got to the Florence station. Once there we looked for the Italia office; we must have looked totally perplexed when a nice man asked us what we were looking for. We said the Italia office and he said, "It is not here." He thought it was a couple stops back on the metro. I did not want to go back and suggested we take our other bags and walk to the hotel nearby where we could calmly sit down and figure this out. We decided to tell our perplexing story to the gentleman at the hotel's front desk-no smirk from him, just a great suggestion to hop a cab for the five minute ride to the other station. It would cost us $10 each way, but it was oh so well worth it. We went up the elevator to our room to unload our other bags, and he would have a cab waiting for us when we came down. Sure enough we made it to the Italia office and we retrieved my purple bag. Now that's the end of that story!

We were still not home though, and more travel snafus ensued. When we were arranging the flights, Kitty had copied my itinerary, but she had missed one detail. Her flight out of Florence was one hour ahead of mine, but we would both lay over in Zurich. Then we were both booked on the same flight from Zurich back to NYC. However there was a delay in my flight taking off in Florence, so my time to make the gate for the departing flight was very tight. My nerves were about shot now, and I kept asking the stewardess if I would make my connecting flight and did she know what gate I needed to get to. No, she did not have that information, but if I was concerned, they would have someone waiting for me when I got off this flight to assist me to get to my departing gate. In Europe, they let you off the plane, and you walk to a bus to take you to the airport terminals. In a crowd of people, there was no one to assist me, so I high-tailed it to the sign designating gates. I had no idea how far my gate was, but I figured I needed to get there ASAP. I was pulling my carry-on bag, and really huffing it. Up escalators made me dizzy, so Kitty and I had been using elevators. Now I felt unstable with the bag and standing on the moving steps, but there was no time to look for elevators. They are very well hidden in airports. I soldiered on, and when I got to the last escalator to my gate, Kitty was standing there pacing, worrying about my making this flight. She was impressed with how I had got there. As for me, I was out of breath and huffing and puffing. Another instance when you think you cannot do something, but you surprise yourself by doing it despite your limitations.

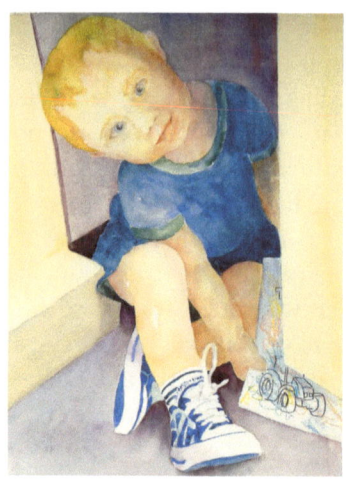

"Nolan peeping" original watercolor

Now Gamma Gail

My reward for making it these fifteen (+) years, is being able to watch my grandchildren thrive. Our oldest daughter Melissa had twins in October 2009. Charlotte and Mason are now 7 years old. When they were first brought out wrapped in blankets by a nurse, I fell to my knees and cried. All the stress of the last few months with monitoring of Mason's heartbeat, (due to the tight quarters) had me always worried. They were both born at least six pounds each. My poor daughter did great throughout the pregnancy considering the weight she was carrying. Having twins is hard and Melissa and then husband Cory struggled, so his mother and I came to stay and help. Feedings initially were rough. Melissa really wanted to breast feed, but Charlotte was a barracuda, and Melissa would cry out in pain. Then Mason did not like to be held that close so she decided to pump, and we would feed them by bottle.

Our younger daughter Megan has a 4-year-old boy named Nolan. He is a spitting image of his dad. Her second son Parker was born December 2015, and she recently had a daughter, Maggie in March of 2017. It is heart-warming to see your child grow as a parent, and Melissa had to learn the hard way with the twins. Having twins is a mixed blessing and I cannot imagine my life without the five of these children. I am glad I was young when I had my daughters, so that I can still keep up with the grandkids on my good days.

Do I Glow in the Dark?

How much radiation can a brain take? I feel like I have reached my maximum between the whole brain radiation, the neck radiation, the Cyberknife and all the scans I have had over the years. Now they are saying I need gamma-knife treatment for a spot behind my right ear. I see two doctors, both radiation oncologists to discuss what they are calling an acoustic neuroma, a cyst that is not on my brain, but pressing on my inner ear nerve. This explains my hearing loss and constant buzzing in my ear. My oncologist recommended I consult with an ENT doctor after he first put me on antibiotics. After a course of that, nothing had changed. The ENT suggested putting a tube in my ear. That has helped, but I still have to consider the gamma knife treatment as the cyst may keep growing and may cause further problems. Our first consult is with a doctor who I just learned yesterday no longer takes our insurance so our costs would be out-of- network. I have been so lucky over the years that my insurance has covered most of our costs and it does cost a lot of money to have the latest drugs. My most expensive treatment so far has been the TDM-1 (Kadcyla) drug that costs $19,000 for an infusion. My insurance covered it all. I really believe having good insurance has kept me alive. This is why I support a local charity, the Cancer Alliance of Help and Hope, Palm Beach County, that gives financial assistance to cancer patients in need of making a co-pay or meeting a deductible or who just needs help with everyday bills. I was on the Board of Directors for over six years and attend their yearly fund-raiser. But this is my first encounter with the worry about what the bill may be. My husband tells me not to worry, and I listen and keep up with my yoga practice and meditation to calm my mind. My heart still goes out to people with high co-pays and deductibles who have to deal with their insurance company on a regular basis. Cancer is hard enough.

Scan Away

Another MRI scan of my brain today. These scans do not get easier to take. The secret for me is to keep my eyes closed once they start moving the bed and keep them closed for the 20 minutes it takes. This time the nurse put a cloth over my eyes and it made it easier to keep them closed. The noise from these machines is deafening, even after they put headphones on you. It is an unrelenting, pounding sound. I just try to concentrate on my breathing and going to my happy place-a hammock overlooking a bay in Hawaii. Yes, I had been in Oahu, staying at a lovely resort. This happy place really exists.

After this MRI they decided to deal with the fluid in my right ear so I had a tube put in at a surgery center. It has helped with the hearing loss I was having. Whether this has anything to do with the spot behind my right ear is a question that may be answered by another scan, this time a Pet/CT. This scan is when they inject you with a radioactive solution, and then you have to sit for 50 minutes and drink a white contrast mixture. You also cannot eat 6 hours prior, so by 10 am I am starving. They throw this warning at you: "Don't be near a baby or a pregnant woman the rest of the day while this solution gets flushed through you." Okay, now I feel comforted.

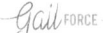

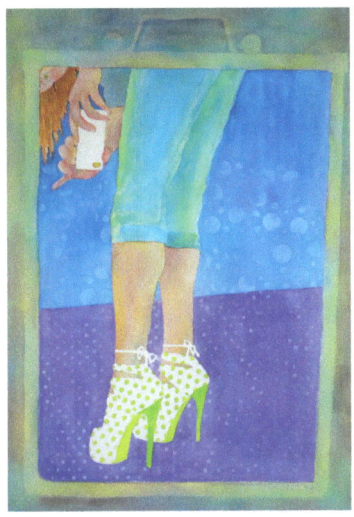

"Selfie" original watercolor

Who Is That Crazy Person?

Another cancer recurrence happened in January of 2015. I had been having pain in my back from the pleurodesis and had seen a pain specialist who gave me pain drugs which made me loopy (or so I thought). I was still walking with my girlfriend in the mornings, and she had begun to notice my speech was slurred. I thought it was the drugs, as did she. Turns out we were both wrong. After a couple of weeks and not adjusting to the pain meds, my speech was getting worse, and I started seeing double. It was time to talk to my oncologists nurse. Immediately, she said I did not sound like myself and I should get a brain MRI that afternoon. My knees felt weak - it must be serious for the urgency of the scan. That evening my oncologist called me and said the scan showed cancer had invaded my brain. That kind of news made the blood drain out of my head. Now I was lightheaded!

My oncologist had me scheduled to see a radiologist on Monday afternoon. The scan was on Friday, I had all weekend to imagine the worst. Believe me those thoughts are hard to shake - no matter how much meditation you do. My husband and I met with the radiologist on that Monday who recommended whole brain radiation, as there were a couple of spots on my brain stem, which they cannot treat with gamma-knife radiation. I was scheduled to undergo the treatments at my local hospital. Ten in all, again with the mesh mask. I did my Dr. Seuss mantra again and imagined a white healing light was killing the cancer. They were short treatments so I barely made it through two mantras. Good news was the radiation worked! My next MRI showed no lesions, and I had just begun a new drug that worked on passing the blood brain barrier. A lot of chemotherapies do not do that, but this drug had just recently been approved, and it worked on my type of cancer-the Her2Nue variety. Science was on my side. Except for a side effect from this drug: my platelets were plummeting. My oncologist changed my treatment to a combo of Xeloda and Tykerb, and I have been on that for eight months now. My major side effect is diarrhea so I have been losing weight. I am trying some supplements to up my appetite and put on weight.

One weekend I went off the deep end and thought I was the "white Oprah." I actually thought I had my own network and was planning jobs for my whole family - no more working for "the man," now they would be working for the "white Oprah." Because of the steroids I had a psychotic episode, and they put me in the hospital on that Monday. Apparently during the weekend I had scared the crap out of my husband who called my oncologist Monday morning.

When we went in for the appointment that day, I was yelling and ranting incoherently. I do not remember any of it - that is the blessing, but my poor husband was traumatized.

When they give you whole brain radiation they also give you steroids, to calm the inflammation. They are horrible drugs and I had a bad reaction to the dose of steroids they were giving me. Because of this reaction to the drugs, I did end up in the hospital again, but this time my oncologist got me a room that overlooked the Intracoastal and Palm Beach, and I could watch the sunrise. It was still a hospital, and the food was horrible, but there are advantages to a good view without the noise of the emergency room. I got to go home on Friday of that week and was so happy, but I was still exhibiting crazy behavior like asking my husband to find my favorite yoga outfit to wear home and to stop and get me a green smoothie. He was not happy making the trip back home. But this was my crazy mind still rearing its ugly head. I rested the rest of the weekend and slowly came back to myself. I felt so bad for my husband because of what he had witnessed. I hope to never have to go through something like that again with any of my loved ones.

They had to strap me down so I would not run away. And my husband had arranged a night nurse to watch me. She was a real stickler for not letting me sit up in bed. At the time, I did not understand. I was getting madder at her as the night went on, but she pretty much ignored me. I could not figure her out. I was complaining about her to my husband when he explained she was there when I was strapped down and she was doing her job to keep me safe. I still did not like her demeanor, but finally broke through her tough exterior when I asked her about her children and her life outside the hospital. Her husband is a pastor of a church so I inquired about gospel music and she invited me to visit. Of course I would be the only white person there (and not being the White Oprah anymore), I would like the courage to go through with visiting, as I do so love a good gospel hymn from my summer Sundays in my mother's hometown Christian church.

I had another MRI of my brain a few weeks later along with a Pet/CT, all still clear! I just made an appointment to have energy work done by an organization called Healing Touch Buddies, a free service to women going through breast cancer, (Visit www.healingtouchinternational.com) Healing Touch is a relaxing, nurturing energy therapy that uses gentle touch to assist in balancing physical, mental, emotional, and spiritual well-being. Healing Touch works with your energy field to support your natural ability to heal, is safe for all ages and works in harmony with standard or allopathic medical care.

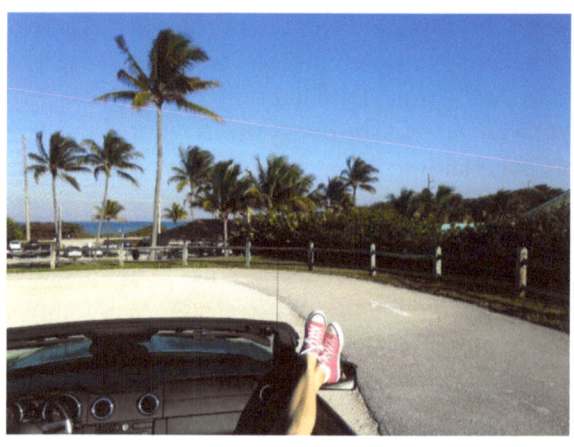

Enjoying a beautiful top down day in Jupiter

Stronger Than Dirt

There used to be a laundry detergent commercial that said, our detergent was "stronger than dirt." People have called me strong for enduring all I have been through with this disease. Do I know where this strength comes from? I feel each time it came back, I was a batter at the plate. I had to do what I had to do to move forward. Be it radiation, chemo, scans, biopsies, I trusted my doctors to a point, but I usually did my homework to understand the options available to me. I am a strong believer in listening to my intuition and asking lots of questions. My faith in God and the power of prayer is my constant companion in this battle. Knowing people were praying for me, gave me the fortitude to fight. I believe in a loving God who does not dole out cancer diagnoses to certain people. I don't believe a loving God would give children cancer and choose who should live or die. Maybe it is what psychologists call "survivor guilt," but why would I live and a child die? I cannot wrap my head around that. I remain humbled by my longevity. "Stronger than dirt." I can embrace the compliment.

Good news, my last three MRI and Pet/CT scans were clear. I met with the radiologist and he says because the tumor behind my ear was stable on the last MRI, he will not be doing anything now. He even said, "I am looking at a healthy brain!" I left his office very happy. So on to making plans with friends and living and breathing and walking - the weather has finally cooled enough.

Basking in that glory did not last long, in April of 2016, my eyes were irritated, lots of pollen here in the Spring, but I had never been affected by it before, and I also had what felt like the shades drawn on my right eye. So I saw an opthamologist who recommended drops, and he diagnosed the darkening as the beginning of glaucoma. The drops did stop the irritation, but the dark shade was still around the top of my right eye. When I called my oncology office to tell them this, they had me seeing a neuro-opthamologist the next day. I had an MRI scan the next morning - now waiting to see the eye doctor again on Wednesday early in the am to avoid the long wait we had on my first visit, than on to my oncologist in the afternoon. "The waiting is the hardest part," to quote Tom Petty.

Moon Dance *(credit Van Morrison)*

After surviving these past (15+) years, the thought of my death has certainly come across my mind many times. I have seen my father die of cancer and friends succumb to this disease. It is not what I would want the end of my life to look like or feel like. But we do not get to choose when the time comes. One of my prayers is to pass in my sleep, as I have said this prayer also about friends and family who are dealing with Alzheimer's, dementia, etc. I do not want to dwell on the end of my life, but it is a butt-kicking reality when the cancer comes back. Maybe my body will reject new treatment, maybe I have too much radiation to have more, maybe science will not be on my side another time.

One thing I am sure in my mind is how I want people to remember me. No funeral parlors, please. I envision a full moonlit night on the shores of the beach in Jupiter, a gathering of family and friends, my playlist softly serenading with my favorite songs. I would like to donate my body to science to help uncover anything science can glean from my physical body to learn more about cancer and the treatments. Cremate my remains and have my family, dig me into the dirt or sand, sprinkle me in the ocean or throw me to the wind. I will not dwell on this any longer. My wishes are known. Amen.

I was on the combo of Xeloda and Tykerb for almost a year; they seemed to be working, so no changes. It is precarious to decide when to stop the chemo, but as long as my tumor markers are stable, I will just keep on soldiering on.

Dark Side of the Moon *(credit Pink Floyd)*

Well, that last bit is no longer true. It has come back in a most troublesome way. It has migrated to my right optic nerve. For a couple of days, I was seeing this dark veil over my right eye, then it went black. I saw my neuro-oncologist who ordered a CT scan of the area and found no tumor but a sheath (they call it a chisam?) enveloping my right optic nerve. Talk about unnerving - this most certainly is and will be permanent. My Onc has put me on Herceptin again, along with 2 tablets of the Tykerb. I was previously taking 4 a day, but the diarrhea was making me lose weight. He was in touch with a DR. out of Duke who formulated this therapy. There is a big cancer conference in Chicago in June of 2016, where he will find out about further studies, possibly immunology.

As of this latest update before publication. I am stable! My Onc. now has me on Xeloda, 2 pills daily, one with breakfast and one after dinner for 7 days then off for 7 days. I'm still on the Herceptin every three weeks.

This has been a good alternative so far, and I continue to thrive and travel and have even added some pounds too. Now my jeans fit better - may not matter to you but, and I mean butt, that's a wrap!

So the story continues hopefully....

*Check out my blog at www.gail-force.com for
further updates or to contact me.*